The Smart & Easy Guide To Relieving Back Pain: The Book Of Natural Treatments, Therapy, Exercises, and Relief For Those Living With Back Pain

Will Jackson

Legal Stuff

COPYRIGHT

LIMITATION OF LIABILITY

Table of Contents

Introduction

As we move through the early years of the new century, the pace of daily life becomes more and more frantic. Every day, there seems to be one more chore, one more task, one more obligation than there was the day before. Modern life being what it is, this breakneck pace will probably just continue to increase. There's not much chance that Wall Street, Congress, the Christmas shopping season, morning rush hour, and MTV will all start to fall back to an earlier, slower pace, even though many people long for a more relaxing time.

As the little stresses on your mind multiply, so do the little physical stresses that affect your body. Unsurprisingly, aches and pains have become such common annoyances that most people don't even bother seeing a doctor about them. Indeed, most people just suffer mutely and hope that their health problems will just smooth out over time.

Most people are so caught up in their hectic daily routine that they avoid even thinking about their back problem. This strategy usually works just fine...until something "minor" slips out of alignment.

Not all pain necessarily demands medical treatment, especially since some pain just comes and goes without any discernible pattern. But not all pain can – or should – be dismissed or ignored. Back pain should always command your attention, even if it seems minor.

Between 50 and 80 million people in the U.S. alone suffer from chronic, or long-term, back pain. Chronic pain is defined as pain that lasts for more than six months. All too often, chronic pain comes in the form of a "bad back." Though sufferers often try to shoo a little long-term backache under the rug, it almost always costs in the end. Believe it or not, when experts calculate the sick time and other factors affected by chronic pain, the cumulative social and economic cost of chronic pain in the U.S. totals more than $100 billion annually.

Backache is also among the most popular reasons for doctors' visits. As many as four out of five people on Earth will see a doctor about their back at some point. It is truly a problem that unites us all. If you haven't already experienced it, then odds are good that you'll know the agony and frustration of back pain at some point in your life. Chronic back pain is on the rise, too. More people than ever suffer from a painful back condition.

If you've never experienced back pain, it's difficult to understand exactly how debilitating it can become. But consider this: your back literally holds up the rest of your body. If your back isn't working right, then your movement will be at least be restricted. If your back bothers you enough, then your every move becomes a trial. Maybe you'll be able to power through it for a while, but how long will you hold up when even picking up a pencil hurts?

The bottom line is this: back pain is awful. Anyone can experience it, but medical science can only do so much to curb the pain and accommodate limitations on mobility. Many back pain victims seek alternative cures in an effort to fill in the gaps in mainstream treatments. Some victims of back pain wish to avoid medication and high medical bills. Luckily, there are a plethora of natural, effective alternative treatments available to for various different kinds of back pain. From massage to acupuncture, there's a remedy for every level and type of back problem.

As with any medical condition, it is safer and often preferable to deal with back pain naturally. Safe, natural back pain relief is the primary topic of this book.

What is back pain?

Putting it simply, back pain happens when you experience discomfort in your back. It is most commonly located in your lower back and usually indicates a problem with the muscles of your back or with your spine.

The biggest problem with back pain is that most people who live with it do just that: live with it. They may be aware that there's something wrong, but hardly give it a moment's thought. The pain isn't acute and there are more pressing matters jostling for their attention anyway.

But as soon as the pain hits, it's immediately Priority #1. There's not much on Earth that will get a person's attention faster than acute back pain. It probably won't matter whether the sufferer is standing, sitting, lying down, or walking. Your back is your support column and when it stops working correctly, so does the rest of your life.

Those lucky enough to suffer back pain intermittently may forget how miserable they were after the pain has gone away. But that's no panacea – the back pain is more than likely to come back without preventative care. Part of the reason for this is that there's no good way to determine what causes most back pain in the first place.

Though lower back pain is one of the leading medical problems in the world, it has too many possible causes to make its treatment easy. From muscle aches to slipped discs, just figuring out why your back hurts can flummox the best doctor or chiropractor for weeks or even longer.

There is good news: for most people, back problems tend to go away on their own. This is called "intermittent back pain" simply because it doesn't stick around. The amount of time you'll need to completely rid yourself of back pain may depend on your condition, the severity of the problem, and so on. But for most people, a "bad back" is ultimately a temporary problem.

That said, once you've had back pain, it's likely to return. That's why even occasional back pain can become a major long-term issue, especially for victims whose job involves heavy lifting. This covers a wide range of surprising professions. Nurses, for example, can suffer major career setbacks if a back problem prevents them from helping heavy patients to sit up. Librarians who need to carry books, shopkeepers who need to carry clothes, and even people who care for children all need to lift in the line of duty, and all can be negatively affected by back pain.

How back pain happens

There are a lot of root causes for back pain, but it all boils down to one rule: almost anything can trigger back pain. There are probably a number of potential back pain triggers already present in your daily life, few of which you could hopr to avoid.

Consider the previous example regarding how nurses must help patients to sit. Back problems are particularly common among members of this profession, and often happen as a result of lifting that they perform in the course of their jobs. One heavy patient can mean the beginning of chronic back pain.

It's common for sufferers of back pain to acquire back problems as a result of their work or lifestyle. Especially tragic is the fact that back pain can be a "side effect" of an otherwise great profession.

Incorrect lifting techniques can also cause back pain. This is because the lower back, which essentially props up your entire upper body, is sensitive to strains and sprains. Those are fairly simple injuries that can happen for a variety of reasons, but especially if you try to lift something by bending your back and trying to use its strength alone to pick up extra weight. It's also fairly common for back problems to start when the victim makes a sudden awkward movement. Suddenly activating out-of-shape back muscles can damage them, especially if they're not accustomed to activity more strenuous than desk work.

Back pain may begin with a single cataclysmic muscle spasm or ramp up slowly. Maybe one area of your back bears too much of your daily stress. If you tax it enough, your back will eventually break under the proverbial straw – or, at least, suffer some serious damage. Ever heard of someone who threw their back out by tying their shoe? Odds are good that the shoe wasn't the real culprit; we have the victim's daily routine to thank for that.

If you wake up one morning and find yourself with some brand-new back pain, review your schedule. Did you do something strenuous the day before? Is there some small. Repetitive movement that you make every day that stresses or strains that part of your aching back? The culprit won't necessarily be obvious. Even sitting at the computer – which may now eat up entire days of the weeks, depending on your profession – can hurt you. Hunching motionless over a tiny screen is as contrary to your spine's natural purpose as lifting a 300 pound box or standing on your hands. If you spend your day at a desk, make sure and move around regularly. Shift your weight and adjust your posture. You could spare yourself a world of pain!

The same goes for anyone who spends a lot of time in the driver's seat. Take breaks, stop for regular strolls, and move around as much as you can while you drive.

Unfortunately, prevention can only go so far. You may find yourself already suffering from back pain, or even coming down with it despite all of your best efforts. If this is your story, then the time to change your routine has passed. For now, focus on getting better. But when the pain fades, resolve to change your habits!

Some back pain is caused by actual medical problems that can only be addressed by an expert. We'll talk more about those in a minute. But intermittent back pain, which tends to come and go on its own, is generally a result of your routine. In other words, if a stiff neck has become a fact of your life, then you're doing something wrong. Time to look over your routine. How do you move? How do you sleep? Most importantly, how do you use – or not use – your back?

Once you've had a chance to analyze your lifestyle, the cause of your back pain will probably reveal itself immediately. Once you find out, don't wait! Prevention is the best cure. As we mentioned previously, doctors struggle to treat back pain effectively. You are in the best position to identify the source of your pain and stop it before it starts.

Of course, while the change you must make may end up being as simple as taking regular breaks, it could also be significant and take much more effort. One major cause of back pain is extra weight. If you're overweight, then your spine is already under too much stress. The likelihood that you'll suffer back pain is much higher. Persistent diet and exercise, as with so many other ailments, are the best prevention.

Time is often the best medicine for back pain. If your pain was caused by an accident, like whiplash often is, then you might have to bear with a long recovery time. In addition to patience, long-term back damage will require medical attention.

There's no way to predict – and usually no way to prevent – random accidents that can hurt your back. But being prepared can still help! Remember, your back pain will only go away so fast. Pushing your recovery will just stall your progress.

What causes back pain

There are a few standard causes that cover most of the back pain that you're likely to ever experience. By far the most common of these are lumbar muscle strains. Most of the back problems that we've already covered fall under this umbrella category. Your lumbar muscles help to support your spine, and when they're hurt, any movement becomes a challenge.

Many athletes are already familiar with the basic concept of a muscular strain. When exposed to a sudden, unusually powerful force, a muscle can tear. Though this is an occupational hazard for a runner or swimmer, anyone who lifts a heavy object too quickly can suffer a strain.

Bad strains become obvious quickly, but minor ones can be hard to pin down. You could just as easily have strained your lumbar muscles by lying down awkwardly as by lifting. It all depends on the stress your muscles are already under.

Luckily, lumbar strains heal quickly and aren't prone to repeat attacks. That's not to say that it'll never happen again, but you probably won't be haunted by the same muscle strain for years.

Back sprains are also relatively common. While a strain is caused by a muscular tear, sprains happen when you overstretch one or more ligaments. As with strains, the ligaments in your back are vulnerable to both immediate and long-term stress. Strains and sprains are treated similarly: lots of rest, mild painkillers, and a review of your routine.

Another popular back problem isn't quite so easy to treat. Disc problems involve the vertebrae in your spine. There are 33 of these running down the center of your back from your head to your hips. If you touch your back, you should be able to feel them as a vertical row of hard bumps. As you can see in the picture, there are four different groups of vertebrae. However, they are all fairly similar in structure.

In between each vertebra, there is a small, soft disc. This disc is made of two parts: an outer coating called the annulus and a firm but flexible center called the nucleus pulposus. These discs act as padding between the vertebrae, enabling your spine to flex without hurting you. This makes your discs critical to everything from walking to lifting your arms. If a disc develops a problem, then your vertebrae may knock together when you try to move. This is extremely painful and limits your mobility greatly.

There are a few disc-related conditions that result in back pain. Of these, slipped disc is one of the most common. A disc slips when the nucleus pulposus, which is the padding inside of the disc, pushes through the disc's surface. There are two possible outcomes to this condition, either of which might or might not be painful. First, you don't have that padding between your vertebrae anymore. Just moving may be much more difficult. Second, the escaped nucleus pulposus sometimes puts pressure on your spinal cord, which is the main nerve in your back, or on other nerves in that area. Anything that goes wrong and involves your nerves is almost guaranteed to hurt.

Slipped discs don't always hurt. The nucleus pulposus might break out without completely deflating your disc. But like many small problems, a minor slipped disc can get worse over time. It's a good idea to see a doctor for this condition whether or not it hurts at the moment.

Having a ruptured disc, which is also called a herniated disc, is much like the condition described above. The difference is mostly semantic; this term usually refers to problems with the cervical and lumbar vertebrae. These five vertebrae do the lion's share of the spine's support work. The ordinary stress on cervical and lumbar vertebrae is tremendous and it's not unusual for the discs in that area to give out.

As we age, our discs become less flexible. Slipped and ruptured discs become more and more likely over time. It's important to be increasingly aware of this common back health hazard.

Unlike many of the other conditions we've discussed, sciatica is a disease. It affects the lower back and sometimes the legs and buttocks. Sciatica is the result of a problem with the large sciatic nerve, which is located in your spinal column. Because sciatica is a nerve problem, it can happen at the same time as a muscular complaint like a strain or sprain, and even at the same time as a slipped disc.

Spinal stenosis also happens more as we age. This condition causes the spaces inside of your spinal column to become narrower. Those spaces house your spinal cord and other nerves, which may experience pressure as a result. As we mentioned before, pain is almost inevitable when your condition affects your nerves. Spinal stenosis is often the result of arthritis.

Osteoporosis is another condition commonly associated with aging, osteoporosis causes bones to become brittle and porous. Because osteoporosis causes bones to weaken gradually, it may cause compression fractures in your vertebrae. This is especially true in the case of elderly and at-risk women.

Though arthritis is most famous for affecting the hands and fingers, it can affect any joint or bone. Lumbar spinal arthritis attacks the backbone. The symptoms are the same as an arthritis sufferer might experience in their hands: difficulty moving, pain, and achiness. Lumbar spinal arthritis can make any movement very painful.

Spondylolisthesis is a much rarer condition. It usually accompanies other degenerative conditions. Adjacent vertebrae become unstable, shifting and grinding together painfully. This condition is painful and frustrating, not only because of its very nature, but because the degenerative disease that causes it is also a priority.

Treating back pain medically

This book focuses on natural back pain solutions, but some problems should always involve a doctor. Something like spondylolisthesis is beyond the ability of natural medicine to cure. Like many serious medical conditions, it must be treated at the source by a trained professional with experience and expertise.

Anti-inflammatory drugs, also known as non-specific anti-inflammatory drugs, are popular prescriptions for many types of back pain. As their name suggests, they reduce the swelling (inflammation) associated with muscular problems. They also reduce pain. Though NSAIDs are considered fairly safe, like all drugs, they have side effects, including gastro-intestinal bleeding and liver stress. Patients who are already taking other drugs that affect their liver and digestive system might want to think twice about taking NSAIDs for back pain.

Narcotic painkillers will reduce some of the symptoms of back pain, but they're also significantly riskier. Many narcotics are potentially addictive and can only be used for a short time.

Your healthcare professional may also prescribe muscle relaxants if the main cause of your back pain is muscular. This drug group includes Valium and other drugs that tend to make you sleepy, if not knock you out completely. Driving and operating heavy machinery is not an option if your medication includes muscle relaxants.

If you're suffering from an inflammation that's located around or near your spinal cord, your doctor might recommend an epidural. This is a steroid injection that reduces pain and inflammation simultaneously. The problems with steroids are fairly notorious. While they can be excellent tools in the hands of a trained medical professional, steroids can't be taken for long periods of time without risk of serious side effects. In this case, you might find yourself only too eager to leave your epidural to memory. Epidurals are notoriously unpleasant experiences that very few people remember fondly.

The rarest solution to back pain is surgery. This is a last resort. Your back is so important and delicate that even excellent surgeons are very reluctant to operate on it. Your doctor will only even consider spinal surgery after every other possible treatment has failed. Only a few conditions are serious surgery candidates, including spondylolisthesis and spinal stenosis. Very, very occasionally, a doctor will operate on a severely ruptured disc.

Most physicians only suggest surgery when the risk of not operating outweighs the danger of your condition. For example, if a slipped or ruptured disc gets no better after a considerable period of non-invasive treatment, it can easily get worse and endanger the rest of your health, never mind your quality of life. A doctor might recommend surgery just to prevent a decline in your condition.

Back surgery is always dangerous, mostly because of the possibility of paralysis. Your spinal cord, which is located in your backbone, gives you control over much of your body. Damaging or stressing that major nerve can be catastrophic. Only consider surgery if the possibility of permanent paralysis is no worse than the possibility of life with your current condition.

Back surgery is extremely rare. Much more common is the natural, home-based treatment of common back pain. We'll talk more about this in the coming chapters. But even if you prefer to treat yourself with ice packs or get a massage, you should know how to choose a doctor if your back problem becomes too much to handle. After all, they are the experts.

When to find a doctor

There's no harm or shame in seeking a professional opinion about your back pain. If your back is bothering you, don't try to "tough it out." You might be glad for the expert attention if it turns out that you have a slipped disc.

As we mentioned previously, the majority of back pain is caused by muscle strain. Though they can be very irritating, muscle strains usually won't require medical attention. Anyway, there's not a lot that your doctor could do for you, aside from prescribing painkillers. Since you're interested in natural cures for your condition, you may not want to use those anyway.

If you can't explain how your back pain began, you might want to go to the doctor for a checkup. This still might not be strictly necessary if the pain isn't acute, but it can be good for your peace of mind.

There are a few specific situations in which you should definitely, absolutely, and immediately seek medical attention for back pain. In these cases, your pain could be a symptom something more serious. Consider any of these symptoms red flags:

• A full week of pain that never abates;

• Inability to control your bowel movements or bladder;

• Flulike symptoms, including chills, hot flashes, and a high fever. These can be signs of a very serious problem and you should see a doctor as soon as possible;

• Any other other unusual symptoms, which is to say, anything that you wouldn't normally associate with a muscle pull.

The problem with back problems

If ask a doctor, you'll learn that diagnosing back pain is among the most difficult tasks in medicine. That's because most back pain looks and feels pretty much the same to both the patient and the doctor. Unless there you already have an established medical condition, like osteoporosis, it's almost impossible for your doctor to pick out the source of your back problem without a slew of tests, scans, and evaluations. Your pain and its location could indicate any number of conditions. In fact, because different people experience pain in different ways, it's sometimes even difficult for a doctor to decide how severe a problem really is. Is it a slipped disc in a patient with a high tolerance for pain? Or a pulled muscle in a patient whose tolerance for pain is low?

If you rarely have back problems, or if you know how you hurt your back, your healthcare provider will have no problem treating you. After all, you already know the cause. In this case, it's probably muscular anyway. Time will do most of the work for you.

But if you live with persistent, long-term back pain, then you might want to consider a different approach. Expecting an accurate medical opinion on your first appointment just isn't realistic. There are too many possible diagnoses. Your healthcare provider will need some time to review your symptoms.

Even if it takes a while to figure out what's going on, avoid "jumping" from doctor to doctor. Nobody is going to come up with an instant miracle cure for your pain. That's all well and good on TV, but it's not the way it works in real life. Instead, find an expert who you like and feel comfortable with. Orthopedists, osteopaths, and some general medical practitioners can treat your back and help you to recover. Once you find a good doctor, expect to work together for several weeks or months.

By sticking with a practitioner, you give them a better chance to discover the source of your problem. Ultimately, you'll get better treatment. Remember, with most back problems, the biggest key to your recovery is time. As many doctors will tell you, being a patient means being patient.

If you find that you're making no progress after a couple months, don't despair. Look into finding a new practitioner.

Rest is the best medicine

To the constant surprise of back pain patients, the most obvious treatment for back pain is also the most effective: rest. This all-natural curative is often as effective for slipped discs as for pulled muscles. Your healthcare provider will probably recommend flat bed rest as the first line of treatment. Don't bend this rule! Defying your doctor's advice will result in setbacks, relapses, and pain, pain, pain. Even if you "feel great" after a few days in bed, don't jump back into your daily life. This is literally the pillar of your health we're talking about. Isn't it worth a few extra days in bed?

Your doctor will probably also prescribe anti-inflammatory drugs and painkillers. If you're more interested in natural treatment, you might not want to take pills. Anyway, medicine can only make you a little more comfortable. You'll still need a ton of downtime to heal. No drug or prescription can prompt your back to repair itself or magically mend overnight. Rest, again, is your ticket to health. Bed rest can also alleviate your pain, especially if you only have a strain or sprain.

That said, avoid staying in bed for more than two or three days. Lying down for so long can start to cause problems of its own, and could even make your original back problem worse.

Now that you know this, you'll understand how carefully you should choose a bed. If you've already had back pain, then your bed may even have contributed to it. A bad bed can make your back problems worse, and bed rest in a bed that's already hurting you is almost a waste of your time. A good bed is a critical investment for anyone with a serious or chronic back problem.

However, this does not necessarily mean that you should invest in a bed that is advertised as "orthopedic." Advertisers often slap this label on mattresses to sell more of them at higher prices, but it doesn't mean that the mattress is actually special in any way. In fact, according to research from the UK, the majority of orthopedic mattresses are too hard. The reputation of orthopedic mattresses is so bad that only 6% of experts recommend orthopedic mattresses to back pain sufferers.

Look for a mattress that is firm and supportive, but not actually hard. It should be comfortable without letting you "sink" into it. Furthermore, if you suffer from chronic or regular back pain, you should think about getting a new bed more frequently. Older mattresses are less likely to give you the support and comfort that your back needs.

If you have some really serious back problems, an argument exists for buying a top-of-the-line bed regardless of the price. The quality of your bed can make a huge difference in the well-being of your back. If you suffer constant back problems, consider spending as much as you can afford on your next bed. All available research seems to suggest that sleeping on a high-quality bed can make a significant difference to your back problems.

Since everyone who suffers a back pain condition has a slightly different problem, there's no single sleeping solution that will apply to every back pain sufferer and ever back condition. That is why you should be ready and willing to do some research when you buy your next bed. Never mind the price – you want a bed that helps to fix your back! That bed could be the difference between your continued, prolonged suffering and the abatement of your back problems.

Also consider the total cost of your back pain in doctors' bills and missed work as opposed to the cost of a bed. If your bed clears up the lion's share of your problem, then you could easily have saved a few thousand dollars at the doctor's. That's not even counting all of the time you lose getting to the doctor, the cost of the medicine you might have to take, and all of the other incidental costs of just being sick. Isn't it worthwhile to splurge on a new bed?

No matter where you live, your local mattress store will offer dozens of choices. Come to the store with a good idea of what you want. Furniture salespeople often work on commission, like car salespeople do, and their attitude can be similar. Don't let yourself be pressured into buying a bed that you don't want, or even worse, a bed that won't help your back!

Test the available mattresses and find ones that feel good to you. A good mattress is not only firm and supportive, but consistent. Lie on your prospective mattress for at least ten minutes. Does it feel as good when you get up as it did when you lay down? Listen to your back! If you're looking at the wrong bed, it'll know.

There are some other small but important points to consider when reviewing mattresses. Is the bed the right height? You should be able to get in and out without any back pain or discomfort. If just getting into bed causes more problems than sleeping on the bed would fix, then that particular bed is not a good option.

Buy the biggest bed you can afford, particularly if you'll be sharing it with your partner. That way, you'll both have plenty of room to move around, get comfortable, and enjoy a good night's sleep.

Finally, take a little time to consider the pillows that you use. How many pillows do you generally sleep with? Do you stack them? If your pillows are piled too high, they could significantly alter the angle of your body – and the position of your back - while you sleep. Resting in an awkward position does your back no favors at the best of times. Your brand-new bed won't help at all if your pillows just make the problem worse.

Think about your sleeping position. The way you sleep right now might be hurting your back anew every single night. Try to find a new position that puts less strain on your back.

Get fit

You've heard this before: prevention is 90% of the cure. Just like with any other medical condition, it's better to take steps against back pain before it hits than to try to treat it once it has developed. You don't need to know the future to expect back pain, either. There are a few conditions that almost guarantee that your back will eventually be hurting. The most significant of these is obesity.

There are a slew of health problems that accompany excess weight. In fact, the list is so long that back pain often takes a back seat to hypertension, heart problems, and diabetes. But back pain is there all the same. If you're overweight, your your spine is already bearing more weight than it naturally would. This means that you're much more likely to experience back problems than you would be if you weighed less. Time to get rid of that extra weight.

The benefits of shedding extra pounds will come back to you threefold. We're primarily discussing the health of your back, but think about all of the physical systems that experience stress and strain as a result of all that weight. Your heart, for example, is undoubtedly under a great deal of stress, your blood pressure suffers as a result of your strained heart, not to mention your increased risk of diabetes.

You've been hearing it for years, maybe decades. While it's annoying to change your lifestyle, the advantages of finally attacking that fat are just too great to ignore. It's never too late! Do your body, your back, and yourself a favor. Spare yourself a major, long-term, obesity-induced back problem.

Working out is almost always a great idea. Even if you're fairly healthy, going to a gym can help you build up extra muscle tone and flexibility. This in turn gives your back the strength to withstand stresses that might otherwise injure it. You'll certainly experience fewer back strains when those muscles are sturdier!

If you're stronger, more flexible, and generally fitter, it will simply be less likely that you'll pull a back muscle and suffer the pain and frustration of a back injury. Plus, you'll feel great! In addition to reducing the likelihood that you'll pull a muscle, exercising has been shown to enhance your body's ability to handle a number of minor medical ailments, including some illnesses. For example, working out can alleviate symptoms of osteoporosis, the degenerative bone disease, long before it develops.

Working prevention into your routine always beats looking for a cure when you're already in pain. This is something that your doctor really can't help with: prevention rests in your hands.

There's no need to become a bodybuilder or weight lifter to reap the advantages of exercise. You don't even need to go to the gym every day. Basic exercises, including walking, tennis, and aerobics, can have a huge positive impact on your health. This is goes double for women. For reasons that medical science still doesn't completely understand, women are at far greater risk of developing osteoporosis than men are. Exercise can be crucial to staving off this heartbreaking condition.

Eating right is beleaguered almost as badly as exercise, but that doesn't change how important it is to your health. A proper diet is just as important to your back health as your regular workout.

One of the biggest long-term factors in your back's health is calcium. If you don't include enough calcium in your diet, the chances that you'll develop osteoporosis skyrockets. Lack of Vitamin D can also increase your probability of experiencing a fracture as you age. Normally, your body will create Vitamin D when your skin comes into contact with sunlight. However, you can bolster your diet with additional Vitamin D if you think that you might not be making enough. Milk often includes added Vitamin D, as do some other common foods.

Also be aware of what you might be taking into your body that isn't helping it. Tobacco and alcohol use can increase your chances of developing back problems in your old age. There are many other documented medical risks associated with these substances, but consider the health of your back just one more reason to quit.

As with most things concerning your health, clean living can head off painful and even crippling medical conditions that are otherwise likely to plague your old age. Remember, osteoporosis weakens your bones, and a broken backbone can mean paralysis. Put in your time now and stop osteoporosis from ever happening!

Not all back problems are muscular

In the course of this book, we focus on muscle pulls and other issues that are often treatable at home. But one back problem that always requires a doctor's attention is a spinal injury. Spinal injuries can be catastrophic. They often result from car crashes, falls, and other traumatic events. An injured spine always means loss of mobility and a long, long road to health. They are often extremely painful, too. Full recovery from a spinal injury isn't always possible.

Initial treatment of spinal injury usually involves surgery to fix the damage manually. Once the surgeons have worked their magic, the job of bringing the injured person back to relative normality is almost always entrusted to healthcare professionals who employ natural means and strategies to do their job.

Some of the strategies that nurses, physical therapists, and caregivers use to care for patients with spinal injuries are useful for anyone with a major back problem. Many can help to reduce back pain significantly, regardless of its source.

Physical therapy: Physical therapists are certified medical professionals whose job is to return injured people to full mobility as quickly as possible. People who have had surgery or other major physical damage will often have physical therapy in the course of their return to health. Physical therapists act as guides and teachers. They will teach their patients specialized exercises and techniques using equipment designed for therapy. If there are any other problems or weaknesses present in a patient's body, a physical therapist will recognize it.

One of the things that a physical therapist might work on with a patient is stretching. Tight muscles and joints can cause a patient to naturally lose mobility. Keeping your muscles limber also decreases the chance that they will become re-injured.

As usual, exercise is a key to back health. If you need an exercise program to strengthen the muscles of your back, then you can find many appropriate exercises on this page.

Aquatherapy: Aquatherapy is also exercise-based. The difference between aquatherapy and working with a physical therapist is that aquatherapy actually occurs in water.

The advantage of exercising in water is that you become weightless. The water supports your body instead of your muscles. You naturally put less strain on your injuries, especially your back. Aquatherapy is a superb way to loosen them and strengthen them in a low-impact environment.

Traction is one therapy method that lends itself well to aquatherapy. Traction is a form of gentle stretching that is particularly helpful for victims of back problems. If you needed traction and opted for aquatherapy, then you might find yourself supported by a float, hanging from your arms, with small weights attached to your legs. This treatment may sound a little strange here, but it works like a charm!

Ultrasound: An ultrasound is a high-energy sound wave. It has many medical uses, from seeing the outline of an unborn baby to repairing damaged muscles and bones to relieving pain. Your medical attendant or physician probably wouldn't recommend ultrasound for a simple muscle strain, but if you have experienced a serious muscular back injury, then it might be a good therapeutic technique.

want to supplement your medical treatment with tried-an
true home cures, consider these alternatives.

As we've already discussed, one simple, effective, and
completely natural way to get rid of your back pain is to s
in bed for a couple of days.

On the other hand, if you already suffer from a chronic ba
problem or fall into a high-risk group, you should conside
making lifestyle changes. Get fit, strong, and healthy befo
back pain strikes! By doing so, you could reduce or elimin
the possibility of back pain forever.

Prevention is a great concept, but if you already have bacl
pain, then you want to know how to get rid of it as quickl
humanly possible. Since you are reading this book, you're
clearly interested in a natural back pain solution. We'll co
alternative back pain treatments over the next few chaptei

The cause of your pain will decide how you treat it. If you
have a serious medical condition, like a fracture, a slipped
disc, or osteoporosis, then treating your back pain at hom
bad idea. At best, you'll waste your time. At worst, you'll
make yourself sicker! Your doctor will be able to give you
best back pain advice and help.

We're going to focus on what you can treat at home: musc
strains, ligament pulls, and other non-critical conditions.
These are annoying, painful, and tend to slow you down.
Luckily, they're also very treatable and respond well to
natural methods.

Remember not to take your back for granted! If your back problem feels too serious to be an easy muscular problem, go to a doctor. The last thing you want is a slipped disc made worse by lack of appropriate treatment.

Heat and ice treatments

Heat and ice are both great treatments for muscular back pain. Your choice as to whether to use heat or ice to treat your back should depend on why your back hurts in the first place.

If you have a back injury, you should first determine whether there's any swelling around the injury. If not, applying heat to your ache is your best option. Heat increases a muscle's flexibility by relaxing it.

If you have to push through your back pain, even if only to get to work and back, heat is likely your best treatment option. Since heat loosens your muscles, you'll find it easier to move around without too much pain.

Heat increases both your blood flow and the temperature of your skin. This means that you're susceptible to burns if you leave heat on your skin for too long. You can safely apply mild heat to your ache for up to 20 minutes at a stretch. Wet heat is most effective, since dry heat can cause your skin to lose moisture, so use a warm, damp towel. Several special heating devices also exist for this purpose, made for athletes with muscle problems. If muscular issues are a hazard of your daily life, then consider investing in one. Many natural heat sources for sore muscles are also available from sources like the National Allergy website.

Sometimes, ice may be a better treatment for your injury. Though heat works well on chronic pain, many other injuries respond much better to cold.

This is especially true when you've suffered from an injury. If you find that your back is swollen or inflamed, ice is your best bet. Low temperature naturally causes causes your blood vessels to constrict, reducing the flow of blood in that area. This stops the internal bleeding that causes your injured muscle to swell.

Wrap ice in a towel before you put it on your skin. This will prevent discomfort and "ice burn." Apply ice to your injured back for up to 15 minutes at once. After that, allow your skin's temperature to come back to normal before reapplying the ice. Repeat this process until your injury feels better.

Ice treatments are a fine home remedy for a little while. After four days, however, consider seeking medical attention. Your problem may be more serious than you can treat solo.

If you hurt your back by performing unusual physical activity or by exercising, then ice treatment may work like a charm. Athletes often use cold treatment to soothe muscles stressed by unusual physical demands.

Both heat and ice treatment can alleviate your pain, soothe your back, and help your muscles to heal. Remember, everyone's body is different. What works for you may not be ideal for your friend. Once you've assessed the problem, decide for yourself whether you would prefer to try heat or cold therapy for your injury.

Many people will try both ice and heat before deciding which one helps more. If you experiment, always try ice first. Heat can make inflammation worse, but ice will alleviate this type of back problem easily without hurting you.

Eating for back pain relief

Many people are surprised to learn how important their diet is to their general health. Athletes have long recognized this fact. Certain foods can help to reduce or alleviate muscle pains, including back pain. Some people argue that the benefits of eating certain foods could be psychological, meaning that they alleviate pain because the person eating believes that the food in question is special. But if it works, then it isn't really important why. The bottom line is that your pain is lessened. Whether the food you're eating has caused a true medical miracle or your mind is just playing tricks on you, your back feels better. That's all that matters!

Sometimes, you may suffer muscle pains in your back because you are experiencing vitamin or mineral deficiencies. This may be especially true if your back pain is a result of a new exercise regime or an activity that you're not used to.

For example, when you sweat, you tend to lose minerals and trace elements from your body. If you don't replace these minerals by including them in your diet, then you could suffer from muscular cramps and aches. Lack of both sodium and potassium can cause problems for your muscles, but both can also be replaced relatively quickly. Sodium is present in most bouillon. Beef or chicken is best, but vegetable bouillon should also work. Bananas are a great source of potassium.

Calcium is crucial not only for your bone health, but for many nervous and muscular functions too. Milk and milk-based dairy products are especially high in calcium, so three glasses of milk a day can replace much of your calcium if you aren't getting enough from other dietary sources. This is particularly true for women who suffer back pain as a result of muscle strains or damage.

Depending on why your back is hurting, even plain water can help. Fluid depletion can cause muscular pain too, and after exercising, you will almost certainly need to replace the water that you have lost by sweating. Even if you haven't been exercising, drinking water can often eliminate or at least reduce back pain. Everyone is supposed to drink at least eight glasses of water every day to maintain good health. If you're not already drinking water, now is the time to start! Your back – and the rest of your body – will thank you.

Back pain, traditional Chinese treatments, and acupuncture

Traditional Chinese medical training does not recognize "simple" backaches: every pain has a systemic cause and effect that impacts the health of your whole body. Moreover, there are several categories into which back pain can fall. Each one must be identified and treated individually.

This is key to understanding popular Chinese medical treatments, especially acupuncture. Acupuncture is roundly acknowledged as a good treatment for back pain, but the specific points upon which a specialist focuses depends on what kind of pain you're suffering from.

Chinese medicine recognizes a number of different back pain types, including the following:

• Deficiency pain usually occurs in middle-aged and elderly people. It's most commonly described as a dull ache. Deficiency pain responds well to rest.

• Blood stagnation is also known as Qi, or "energy flow," pain. Qi is energy that saturates the body and allows it to function properly. Traditional Chinese medicine holds that muscles can move this energy, along with blood and other bodily fluids, by stretching. If your muscles don't work enough, your Qi becomes congested, sticking in your muscles and making them hurt. Significant or even serious pain can result. In our desk-bound, all-too-often sedentary society, your Qi is constantly in danger of becoming congested.

• On chilly mornings, some back pain patients might experience cold and damp obstruction pain. Cold and damp weather tends to make this type of back pain worse. Western medicine often associates cold and damp obstruction pain with arthritis, sciatica, and similar conditions. Because of that, this type of pain often includes the other symptoms of those diseases. Numbness, heaviness, and swollen back muscles often accompany back pain of this type. Heat is the best treatment.

Chinese medicine has it that pain and discomfort are messages from your body. Your physical balance has somehow been upset and must be corrected. You won't get relief until your internal order has been restored. Acupuncture is among the best ways to bring harmony back to your body.

Today, acupuncture assumes that most of us don't use our muscles enough. We sit for long hours, often close to completely still, watching TV or using computers. As a result, we don't stretch and contract our muscles. Our muscles become tight and cramped, stopping Qi from flowing naturally through our bodies. When we do try to use our muscles, the balance of Qi is so poor that even little movements can throw a muscle into a spasm. Because the back already bears most of the weight of your body, the muscles there are most susceptible. If your Qi is blocked, then even something as simple as bending over to pick something up from the floor or brushing your teeth can immobilize you.

An acupuncturist will use needles to move blood and Qi around your body. A trained acupuncturist knows the many different blood and Qi "channels" in your body. Their first task will be to palpitate different parts of your back to establish the locations of your most serious problem areas. These are your "points of pain."

Points of pain are places where Qi has become congested. The more pain there is, the more congestion exists in that spot. In order to treat this congestion, the acupuncturist will insert needles into your body to open your Qi channels and release the congestion. This will help to remove your pain.

Your acupuncture practitioner will apply needles at both local and distal points on your body. Local points are actually located at the site of the pain that you feel. There are many points on the back itself where the insertion of needles can be very helpful. Distal points are located in other parts of the body, but are connected to the pain through Qi channels. Although the acupuncturist's method may appear to be somewhat counterintuitive, distal acupuncture points are critical to effective acupuncture. This is especially true if your back pain is acute. Even if your practitioner places needles a considerable distance from your pain, this method can be very effective.

If you're not enthusiastic about needles, there are alternatives available. Some practitioners use an electric current instead of needles to stimulate the flow of your Qi. This method eliminates the need for needles altogether, and many people who would otherwise avoid acupuncture prefer this modern method.

Many people unfamiliar with acupuncture may question the possible benefits of this ancient method. Does acupuncture work as a treatment for back pain? In 2002, two leading Swedish doctors undertook a clinical study to determine the answer to exactly this question. The results appear to be an unqualified "yes." Acupuncture works!

According to the results published in "The Clinical Journal of Pain" and reported on the Acupuncture Today website, the two researchers tested acupuncture using a group of people who had been suffering from chronic lower back pain for at least six months. Every one of these people had tried various other back pain relief treatments or cures without seeing any improvement in their condition.

The test group was split into three smaller groups. Test subjects in the first subgroup received traditional acupuncture treatments every week for eight weeks. In the second group, subjects received electro-acupuncture, the needle-free alternative that we explored above. Members of the third subgroup were given a placebo.

The final results of the test indicated that all of the patients who had received acupuncture reported "significant" improvement in their condition as reported one month, three months, and six months after they had completed the treatment. They also reported that they were able to sleep more soundly and enjoy higher activity levels than they had prior to the study. There is little doubt that acupuncture is an effective treatment for back pain.

The test also reported that certain types of back pain and patients responded to treatment better than others. Perhaps most interestingly, the study indicated that both traditional and electric acupuncture were equally effective. This is great news for people who simply can't stand needles! Thanks to modern technology, acupuncture is now for everyone.

This study also examined use of the local and distal points that we discussed earlier. Though many people find this system particularly counterintuitive, it nevertheless came through well for the participants. These are the points of the body where acupuncture was used during the 2002 Swedish study.

Chiropractic manipulation

Chiropractors can be tremendously helpful in relieving back pain, too. Experts in back pain, chiropractors can effectively manipulate your muscles back to health.

Indeed, chiropractic manipulation can in certain circumstances be every bit as effective as medical treatment for a back pain condition. That is, going to a chiropractor can sometimes be as effective as getting a prescription from a doctor!

However, it is extremely important to understand that chiropractic manipulation is not ideal for every situation. Sometimes, it can even make your back problem considerably worse. It all depends on why your back is hurting. For example, if your back pain is a result of spinal damage, then chiropractic treatment can be extremely dangerous.

In order to prevent problems from arising in the chiropractor's office, make sure to get an x-ray before you visit the chiropractor. This will help you to establish whether you have any spinal damage or instability. Your chiropractor will be as relieved as you are to know what's causing your pain.

Also seek mainstream medical attention if you have pain in other areas, especially in your buttocks or legs. This could indicate other medical problems that a chiropractor couldn't treat. Numbness or tingling is also a warning sign of more severe conditions, and you should seek a doctor before considering visiting a chiropractor for treatment.

Massage for back pain

Many people find that a good massage will help to alleviate their back pain. However, this relief is often relatively temporary. It can be valuable if it is the only treatment that affects your pain, but expect to make regular visits to the masseur. If your pain is serious enough, then the only thing you have to lose is the money that you'll pay.

The same precautions apply to the masseur as applied to the chiropractor. Make sure and find out why your back is hurting before you take any other action! A masseur could make certain conditions worse while intending to help.

Herbs for back pain

Current research suggests that depression and stressful events can make pain worse. Sufferers of chronic pain are likely to experience greater physical agony if they also come down with depression or succumb to stress. This research goes on to suggest that substances that calm and soothe your nervous system will also help to relieve your pain.

Stress-reducing herbs can be crucial allies in your fight against back pain. There are many herbal remedies for stress, many of which also help treat depression and insomnia. Skullcap can be a very helpful stress treatment; as can valerian root, which is a popular sleep aid; St John's wort; poppy, which is the source of morphine; willow bark, which is the source of aspirin; cayenne, the same substance as the popular red cooking spice; wild yam; angelica; motherwort; rose; and lavender.

In addition, essential oils extracted from pine, peppermint, rosemary, ginger, frankincense, cloves or juniper can all act as natural painkillers. Add between 10 and 12 drops of essential oils from any of these herbs to one liquid ounce of olive oil or coconut oil. Shake the mixture well and rub the oil on the painful part of your back. This will both help to alleviate the pain and reduce swelling.

If you live with chronic back pain, try drinking a few cups of skullcap infusion every day. You could alternatively try taking a dozen or so drops of skullcap tincture every day. If you want to try something else, a mixture of skullcap tincture, St John's wort and oat straw in equal parts can calm the nerves, which will can in turn lessen the pain in your back.

St John's wort oil can be liberally rubbed on any part of your back that hurts, and since it's a very powerful treatment for muscular pain, this can be a great way to safely treat chronic or acute muscular back pain.

Yoga to deal with back pain

Contrary to popular belief, yoga is not a form of exercise. Nor is it about striking poses. Yoga's real purpose is to teach devotees to adopt a totally balanced approach to life, covering both physical exercise and mental adaptability.

Most importantly for any back pain sufferer, yoga puts great emphasis on the physical alignment of your body. Misalignment of the spine and poor posture are among the top causes of back pain, so yoga can be a tremendously useful preventative technique.

If you spend many hours sitting at your desk every day, work at a computer, or drive professionally, then you are almost definitely putting your back in a stressful position. You may not experience a single traumatic event that causes all of your back pain, but over time, your constant sitting position will make back problems almost inevitable. Now might be a good time to try yoga!

Yoga is ideal for alleviating back pain. In the first place, because yoga places a great deal of emphasis on spiritual practice that demands the practice of controlled breathing. Controlled breathing, also called pranayama, naturally relaxes your muscles. This relaxation reduces the chances that you will suffer a muscle strain or sprain in the first place, but if you already have an injury, relaxation will help to alleviate the pain.

Yoga poses, also called asanas, are all about stretching. Remember, your muscles are more vulnerable to injury when they aren't limber and flexible. When you practice Yoga, you work your muscles enough to make sure that they won't strain or sprain during everyday activity.

Yoga can help to maintain your back's health in a couple of different ways. First of all, it can reduce your pain. Loosening your muscular tension can greatly reduce the consequences of a sprain or a strain. Second, keeping your back flexible can also prevent back problems from developing. If your body is already used to moving around, it's less likely to give way when you make demands of it during the course of your daily life.

The fact is this: if you do not already take regular exercise, whether that is a morning jog, a brisk swim, a bicycle ride around the park or even a walk in the local nature preserve, your spine will have become more rigid and less flexible. That is simply a recipe for pain. Without regular stretching workouts, and use, your back simply won't be ready to withstand injury when it encounters stress.

That said, taking up a strenuous activity can be bad for your back too. Aggressive athleticism is all too often the cause of back injuries. Yoga is the perfect solution: it allows you to strengthen your back, improve your flexibility, and avoid serious injury. It is low-impact and relaxing. Even jogging is relatively stressful to your body – think of your feet pound-pound-pounding on the sidewalk hundreds of times per mile. That activity can easily trigger lower back problems. Yoga includes no such risk.

Nevertheless, if you are thinking of taking up yoga either to alleviate existing back pain or to prevent a future back pain problem, you should consult your healthcare professional. While Yoga isn't as immediately stressful as, say, football, it is nevertheless exercise, and you should have medical confirmation that you're up to the task before embarking on yogic training.

It's also a good idea to start training under the professional supervision of a qualified yoga teacher. While many websites feature illustrations of back-friendly positions, never try them alone, no matter how easy they look. Yoga is a complicated form of exercise that takes years to master. At worst, you could injure yourself; at best, you won't see the benefits. It's safer and probably more productive to learn these poses from an expert.

This is true even of poses that look easy. The "Balasana" pose, which is also called the "Child pose," is commonly recommended to sufferers of back pain. Here's an image from the Yoga cards website:

Looks simple, right? Though this position may seem straightforward, there are subtleties present that only a professional can explain. When the simple act of bending over can throw your back out, why take the risk of teaching yourself yoga? Find a good trainer and enjoy your yoga instruction safely.

Once you begin studying yoga, you'll run into a number of great websites devoted to this practice. In addition to the yoga cards site whose graphic is featured above, you might also want to look at articles about yoga and back pain on about.com, study some of the recommended poses from the same site, and read about back pain relief extracts from 'Yoga for Wellness' here.

Conclusion

As we've discussed in this book, there are many ways to deal with back pain without resorting to pharmaceutical chemicals or drugs. Simple at-home treatments, lifestyle changes, and exercise can all work wonders on your chronic or acute back problem. When you consider your back pain, consider also making adjustments to cope with it. Even if it means shoehorning half an hour of stretches into your busy morning routine, it's worth it! Wouldn't you rather do a little extra work to avoid the crippling agony of a strained back?

The most important thing to take away from this book is that treating your back pain can and should be a natural process. There is no need for your back pain treatment to be difficult. It's hard to imagine anything simpler or more natural than sleeping in a comfortable bed.

Personally, I thoroughly recommend yoga. Anyone who suffers from back pain can benefit, and the preventative powers of yoga are amazing. Once you learn, you can practice in private, in classes, at home, whenever you feel like it, or whenever you have a free moment. For the price of a few introductory yoga classes, your back pain can become a thing of the past.

Now that you've completed this book, managing your back pain naturally should be easy. No matter what method you use, make sure to remember that you're not just doing this for your general health: you're guaranteeing your ability to move and function for the rest of your life!

All that's left is to put it into practice. You CAN manage your back pain naturally! Review this book for tips and make sure to consult experts when you need to. Take control of your back back pain today!

We Want Your Feedback on This Book!

Our main purpose is to make sure that our readers get value from the books we publish and that they have a good experience with all of our products. We are always working to improve our books and other products with every revision and update.

Every piece of feedback makes a difference in this process. And we would appreciate yours as well - whether it is good or bad.

Please take one minute to let us know what you thought by following this link:

http://checkmatemg.com/feedbackbackpain